CAROLE MAGGIO

FACERCISE

CAROLE MAGGIO

FACERCISE

The Dynamic Muscle Toning Programme
for Renewed Vitality and a
More Youthful Appearance

BY CAROLE MAGGIO
WITH KYLE RODERICK

B🌿XTREE

First published in Great Britain 1995 by Boxtree Ltd

This edition published 1996 by Boxtree
an imprint of Macmillan Publishers Ltd
20 New Wharf Road, London N1 9RR
Basingstoke and Oxford
Associated companies throughout the world
www.macmillan.co.uk

ISBN 0 7522 0566 8

7 9 8

A CIP catalogue record for this book is available from
the British Library.

Printed and bound in Great Britain by
The Bath Press, Bath

This book is dedicated to my dear friend, Joan Christensen. Without her unending support this book would not have been written. To my sister Michal, who pushed me to continue to share my dream and to Gloria, whose "vision" always inspired me to help others achieve their dreams.

CONTENTS

INTRODUCTION 9

INTRODUCTION

All attractive women share the same beauty secret: they care enough to make the best of their unique features. Although there are few things in this world that we can control, you *can* control how well you look, if you're willing to make the effort. This book is a key to your self-improvement efforts.

I have successfully taught Facercise for more than ten years to hundreds of clients across the United States, England, France, Brunei, Hong Kong, Singapore, Jordan and Japan. Facercise will teach you the skills to help you recapture and maintain a younger, healthier and more vital-looking face.

Facercise is a natural approach to reshaping your facial appearance. When devising the exercises, I consulted plastic surgeons and other doctors to ensure their safety and effectiveness. By carefully following the Facercise programme, you can strengthen and develop the facial muscles so that the face is actually restructured to achieve an improved, younger look. With Facercise, you can take ten years off your face, without silicone, stitches or surgery. All you have to do is work your facial muscles.

Just as a body builder develops his or her physique by isolating and working muscles one by one, you can accentuate or develop cheeks, lips, the eye area, and other facial features by repeating a specific exercise. Because the muscles in the face are so small and responsive, dramatic results can be achieved quickly, sometimes in a matter of hours.

By working out the facial muscles underneath the skin, you tone and tighten up the underlying structure of your face. Performing Facercise properly also increases the blood circulation in the skin, so pale or sallow complexions become peachy-pink and glowing. The overall result is a firmly toned, rosier face; within three days, there is usually a noticeable improvement in the facial contours and complexion.

To understand the benefits that you will enjoy from Facercise, let's first consider how the face ages. We have fifty-seven facial muscles, most of which we rarely work. As you age, muscles flatten and elongate with lack of use and the pull of gravity; sagging skin is the inevitable result. As time passes, the bone, muscle and fat under the facial skin – and elsewhere on the body – actually diminishes while, at the same time, the skin loses its elasticity. By now, most of us are aware that sunbathing and environmental stress causes wrinkles, but habitual facial movements – such as furrowing your brow and squinting when you're confused – can also etch lines into your skin.

ULTIMATE CONTROL

Although surgery can pull the skin tight across the face and lift it up, the elements that cause wrinkles and sags still remain and will ultimately prevail. In time, the same wrinkles and sags that were present before surgery reappear to varying degrees.

Whereas plastic surgery deals with the symptoms of ageing skin, Facercise deals with some of the causes: weakened underlying muscle and constricted blood circulation in the face. While a surgical facelift can offer visible results, it's an expensive and painful procedure with short-lived benefits. Facelifts routinely require follow-up surgery after several years and, with each additional surgery, the face often appears more tightly stretched. Facelifted faces can appear hard and mask-like – anything but youthful. Many people who sign on for plastic surgery eventually find themselves too gravity-stricken or age-afraid to get off the merry-go-round.

For far less money and discomfort than plastic surgery entails, Facercise provides natural, long-term results that are more appealing. Instead of putting your destiny in the hands of a plastic surgeon, Facercise empowers you by giving you ultimate control over your face. This programme will give your looks a lift without scars (or having to wear eyebrows in the middle of your forehead, like some plastic surgery veterans I've seen).

Facercise is not a one-time procedure but a continuing improvement programme. Be patient, read the exercise instructions closely and practise. Once you've mastered the Facercise exercises, you can do them anywhere, anytime – in the car, on the phone, while you're doing the housework or sitting at a computer.

Do your Facercise exercises properly and you will continue to improve your appearance every week, every month and, as the years go by, just how youthful you grow is up to you!

①

HELP YOUR FACE!

My fascination with beauty began in, of all places, a lift. I was fourteen years' old at the time, and was standing beside my mother when a woman with a strange-looking, unnaturally tight face stepped in. I couldn't take my eyes off her. When we got out of the lift, I asked my mother, 'What on earth was wrong with that woman's face?'

'She's had a facelift, Carole,' she said. 'You know, they call it plastic surgery.'

That woman in the lift was someone I determined never to look like. I instinctively felt that her facelift achieved the opposite effect of a beautiful face. I believe that looking as good as possible is part of living a full and happy life, but I also know there are many roads to beauty. I've always been concerned with my looks, and I have always cared very much how other women look. I love seeing a woman look her very best.

In my early twenties I became an estate agent, got married and had a family, and my avid interest in beauty became an active hobby. I read everything I could on the subject, from beauty magazines to medical books; I studied and kept files. This research into the art of skin care, with a special interest in anti-ageing treatments and cosmetics, led ultimately to a career change.

Within six years, I became a qualified beauty therapist and opened a skin and figure salon in Monterey, California. At that time I myself was combating two common beauty flaws: cellulite and dry, lined skin from too many years of suntanning. I knew that if I needed help with these problems, then other women probably did, too. The salon was a great success, and it gave me the valuable experience of working with many different women. I learned to see how a woman's face becomes a map of her habits, her emotional history and her state of mind. And I learned how to enhance each woman's unique beauty.

INSPIRATION

In the seven years that I ran my salon, I refined my knowledge of the latest and most touted beauty treatments. I flew around the world to take classes with the foremost professionals in the field. I trained with Beverly Hills skin care experts and medical doctors to acquire new information and expertise. Dr Gerald Snyder taught me hand-lift massage, a wonderful skill to master. The massage tones the skin and increases blood circulation so much that it made my clients look like they had just had a facelift. Although this massage was extremely effective, the 'facelift' only lasts a week. Still, my clients felt wonderful and looked better as each week of treatment went by.

I used a variety of skin care regimes in the salon. At one time I was carrying products from nine different companies because I couldn't find any one that offered all the results I sought.

By the time I was thirty-six, the fine lines on my face were growing more visible – and more difficult to fill out. Although I performed anti-ageing treatments such as lymphatic drainage and hand-lift massage in my salon, I could not perform these methods on myself. And none of my employees could do them because the techniques were too specialized. Imagine my frustration: I could work wonders for my clients but was incapable of improving my own appearance.

Around this time my husband, who is sixteen years my senior, casually mentioned that he thought I was looking my age. I was devastated. But I knew he was right. The good news is that his remark made me take stock of my situation – and then my inspiration came. I realized that if I could somehow plump up the underlying structure of my face, the lines would fill out and diminish. My face would appear smoother and more toned.

I began to study the anatomy of the face and to learn how the facial muscles work. I read textbooks on the theory of exercise, and I studied and experimented until I knew how to isolate and manipulate the major muscles in my face. Slowly and carefully, I began to develop an exercise programme that would 'recontour' my face the way I wanted it to look.

I worked away in secret. After about six weeks of 'working out', one of my regular clients confronted me and said accusingly, 'What are you doing to your face? You look younger.' I confided that I had been creating and practising facial exercises. She was so impressed with the positive changes she saw in my face, she said, 'Teach me how to work out the same way.' I explained that I wasn't sure I could teach anyone what I'd been doing in private – after all, the exercises were something that I had been refining for myself, on myself – but I'd be happy to give her face a try.

If only I had taken a picture of this woman before we began working together. I had no idea how rapidly I could teach her to develop the muscles of her face. I devised a twenty-minute daily programme for her and, to our mutual delight, her appearance changed dramatically in just five days.

MY CLIENTS

Six days after we first started working together, she asked me to take a Polaroid snapshot, and the next day she brought in a photo that had been taken three years before. When we placed the photos side by side, the difference was strikingly obvious. Not only did her face look younger, well-toned and rosier, but there was a new light in her eyes. The exercises had increased circulation and oxygen flow in the muscles around her eyes, and they were sparkling. This woman sent me the first of many client letters thanking me for the great improvements I had made in their appearances. (I've included some other testimonials at the back of the book – look for them after Chapter 6.)

I felt quite touched by the gratitude of my first Facercise client, but I reminded her, 'I may have given you the tools, but you did the work. Thank yourself.' And I meant it. This wonderful lady committed herself to working on her face and she looked fantastic.

She deserved to feel proud. This success with my first Facercise client led me to the conclusion that if people are willing to spend hours each week exercising their bodies, then they should be willing to give their faces a few minutes a day, too.

I was right, and word of mouth about my exercises spread quickly. After achieving similarly dramatic improvements with clients of all ages, I acquired a professional understanding of how different faces age and how they can be revitalized by working the muscles underneath.

Through working with various women – and a few men – I learned how to raise the eyebrows, shorten noses, enlarge lips, plump up cheeks and tighten jawlines and triple chins. I also grew to see how, as the years go by, we naturally lose the fat cells in the face. Our bones shrink, and the ageing face can take on a more brittle or sagging look. I even noticed – and later read medical documentation confirming my observation – that the nose lengthens throughout life. It never stops growing! As I saw people benefit from my facial exercises, I envisioned how every face, regardless of age, shape, or texture, could derive anti-ageing benefits from a custom-designed exercise programme – and thus Facercise was born! And Facercise delivered a bonus beauty treatment: the exercises themselves proved to be stress-relievers. Facercise would wage battle on frown lines, angry mouths and worry lines on two fronts!

As my Facercise business grew, I continued to research the benefits and drawbacks of cosmetic surgery. I realized that for some people, successful cosmetic surgery can rejuvenate their looks and polish their self-image and confidence. But plastic surgery may not be the answer for everyone. A facelift stretches and pulls the skin and muscles back to the ears; it can emphasize the ageing, brittle look of one's features. I'm talking about the same artificially tight look that I first saw in the lady in the lift when I was fourteen.

I know there are some surgeons who are masters of reconstruction and beautification. To find a good one always involves research, and the more research you do, the better the chance you'll find an artist–surgeon. You must start by collecting referrals from satisfied patients, then you can interview doctors and look at photographs of their work before you make any decisions.

The most enlightened doctors realize that there are important adjuncts to plastic surgery such as customized skin care and facial exercises. Many plastic surgeons refer their patients to me because they know that Facercise can help construct and reshape muscles weakened from facelifts and other surgical modifications. When done properly, Facercise strengthens the muscles and helps maintain the beneficial looks of plastic surgery.

About 60 percent of my clients are people who have had some form of plastic surgery – an eyelift, a rhinoplasty or a complete facelift. Not all of these surgeries were successful, and I can sympathize with people who are disappointed with their cosmetic surgery as I had a bad nose job that left a dent on the left side of my nose. Yet Facercise helped shorten my nose tip (it was left too long) and fill out the dent. Now it's invisible.

Many of my clients who have had cosmetic surgery are determined not to go back for follow-up operations five to seven years down the road. In that first year after surgery, I teach them to exercise and build up the facial muscles to prevent the need for subsequent maintenance operations. Facercise gives them good results and a sense of control over their own destinies.

While I'm not opposed to cosmetic surgery, it's worth noting that there is always an element of risk involved. Even the greatest surgeons can fail to deliver the results they promise. Health, age and skin elasticity all influence how the face will respond to surgery. There are so many variables to be considered, whereas with facial exercises, the process is risk-free and results are predictably beneficial. By learning how to pump your facial muscles, you will nourish every cell in your face with life-giving blood.

TRIUMPHS

A natural alternative to surgical intervention, Facercise provides a gentle and ever-renewable way for an individual to triumph over his or her genetic destiny. (Many of my clients come to me when their mouths start to look like those of their mothers!) Facercise helps reinvent a younger, more relaxed-looking face. After a single session with one of my clients, she told me, 'I've been looking for someone like you for ten years! Now there's no need to resort to a facelift!'

My clients range in age from twenty to eighty-seven. My eighty-seven-year-old is an energetic lady who loves tap dancing and since her Facercise training looks as young as she feels. Many of my younger clients are already veterans of unsuccessful plastic surgeries, and the older ones enjoy a vital shot of self-esteem by 'lifting' their faces with Facercise. Experience has shown me that you're never really too old – or too young – to start Facercise.

Some of my most interesting clients are people who use Facercise to help overcome physiological damage sustained from paralyzing illnesses or disfiguring car accidents. I once trained a man in his fifties who had been stricken decades before with Bell's palsy, a condition which had paralyzed one side of his face and partially closed an eye. From the very first session he threw himself into his exercises, despite his disability. By the second afternoon he started regaining feeling in his formerly paralyzed facial muscles. His eyes filled with tears.

'Carole,' he said, his voice breaking with emotion, 'after thirty-five years I have feeling in my face – the numbness is gone. Thank you for helping me in a way that no doctor ever has.'

It intrigues me whenever I read or hear an interview with a dermatologist or a plastic surgeon on the subject of facial exercises. Those who know nothing about it will make a statement to the effect that there is no scientific proof that facial exercises are effective in recontouring the face. Yet some of the world's leading medical authorities have gone on record in favour of facial exercises.

CAREER HIGHLIGHTS

According to Dr Wilma Bergfield, the President of the American Academy of Dermatology, 'Exercising facial muscles in a reasonable fashion certainly can improve the general appearance of the skin's surface without harming it in any way.' Many physicians also see the therapeutic value of Facercise. Dr Lawrence Birnbaum, a Beverly Hills plastic surgeon, says, 'The exercises as taught by Ms Maggio are extremely beneficial to both pre- and post-operative cosmetic surgery patients. They can also help anyone else lift sagging facial skin via building up the fifty-seven facial muscles.'

After a few years of teaching Facercise in the United States, my business began to blossom all over the world. I've taught international celebrities and business leaders, and I've been summoned by movie stars to film sets the day they're shooting close-ups. My career highlights include giving Facercise seminars for beauty professionals at the University of London and at Les

Nouvelles Esthetiques Congresses in France and England. In 1994 I addressed the Beauty and Health Conference in Hong Kong, and a few months later the British women's magazine *Harpers & Queen* and the Italian fashion house Emporio Armani invited me to speak at a glamorous charity benefit they sponsored.

WHAT FACERCISE CAN DO FOR YOU

I have been teaching Facercise for more then ten years now, and I am continuously refining, expanding and updating the exercises. Although I first started doing the exercises with women, today about a quarter of my clients are men. My male clients include Hollywood actors, business executives, British rock stars, and Middle Eastern royalty.

Facercise is tailored to enhance and maintain individual facial features, but I want to stress that you don't have to do the whole twenty-minute programme in one sitting. It's a flexible, adaptable routine whose exercises can be easily merged into your day. For example, you can do your eye exercises while talking on the phone or while you wait to pick up your kids from school. Do your nose exercises while you read during your lunch hour. I have even tailored all of the exercises so that they can be done while driving the car.

Facercise is just about the most user-friendly health and beauty regime ever invented. Consider this book a personal trainer for your face, and your mirror will provide progress reports.

I take photographs of new clients before they begin the programme and then a few days later. I have hundreds of these photos I've collected over the years. The camera never lies. Changes are visible in a photograph after just a few days of doing Facercise for twenty minutes a day. Those who devote twenty minutes a day to the exercises for at least five days a week often see results greater than ever hoped for other than by surgery. The pictures are proof. (You'll find some in Chapter 3.)

I want my clients to understand how Facercise will help them in ways that plastic surgery cannot. That's why I discuss with them the perils and possibilities of ageing faces. Although gravity pulls your face down as you age, Facercise can help you counteract this. And, although Facercise will make your face look more toned, it can't restore collagen, the connective fibres in skin that give it elasticity. Unfortunately, nothing can restore collagen as you age.

Here's the briefing I give to all my clients regarding what happens to your face as it ages:

❑ Skin tone grows pale or yellow
❑ Nose continues to grow longer and/or wider
❑ Lips grow thinner
❑ Eyebrows and eyelids droop
❑ Under-eye puffiness increases
❑ Jawline sags and jowls develop
❑ Mouth corners sag or turn down
❑ Chin sags; double chin can develop
❑ Skin on neck grows loose and crêpey

The good news is that by doing the exercises in this book, you can expect the following results:

❑ Rosier skin tone
❑ Raised or lifted eyebrows
❑ Enlarged eye sockets, making eyes look more open
❑ Diminished puffiness under the eyes
❑ A shorter or narrower nose
❑ Fuller lips
❑ Firm jawline, diminished jowls
❑ Turned-up, young-looking mouth corners
❑ Toned and smoothed chin and neck

In addition, increased blood circulation and oxygen flow throughout the skin and facial muscles will bring about a rapid improvement in skin colour. Sallow, yellow skin, or chalky-white complexions will change to fresh, glowing rosy tones. In my experience, the skin tone transformations are most notable in Asian faces that are yellowish-grey. (My work in Tokyo has been especially exciting because Japanese complexions bloom so quickly.)

Facercise has brought me profound professional and personal fulfilment and it's a pleasure to share my programme with you. If you read this book carefully and do the exercises properly, you will see and feel great changes in your face and vitality. Ultimately, Facercise will benefit body and soul. Remember that your mind can make your face more beautiful. Now that's what I call powerful!

$$\textcircled{2}$$

WHAT IS FACERCISE?

How and why it works

Like me, you've probably looked at people's faces all your life and said to yourself, 'That woman is blessed with good bone structure,' or, 'She has great cheekbones, no wonder she's so beautiful.' Of course, good bone structure is a key component of facial beauty, but few people realize what an important role facial muscles play in moulding the contours of the face. Do you realize that without facial muscles, you could never smile, blink, or frown? Nor could you sneeze, laugh or yawn.

Muscles in the face are smaller and thinner than most other muscles in the body. But because the fat-to-muscle ratio in the face is lower than it is in most other parts of the body, developed facial muscles can become quite visible, giving your face a firmer and more finely sculpted appearance. I've seen dramatic results achieved in a much shorter time than it takes for changes to appear in, say, the thighs or stomach.

Facial muscles are terribly under-used: people exercise their bodies, not their faces. Naturally, it follows that most people have weak facial muscles, which invariably sag. And when the muscles sag, the skin attached to them also sags. (You know what an upper arm with an undeveloped triceps looks like.) In fact, slack facial muscles are one of the main causes of the sagging and drooping that most of us eventually experience.

YOUR MUSCLES

Sagging is a result of the inevitable reduction in collagen and elastin – the skin's connective fibres – as we age. These fibres give skin elasticity and suppleness, and there's no way to restore these substances. Shrinkage of diminished subcutaneous fat (fat under the skin) also contributes to sagging. Fat reserves under the skin grow smaller with age, and this can partially account for that mid-life 'gaunt' look that hollows out an ageing face.

Sagging produces bags under the eyes, loose folds of skin on the upper eyelids, pouches, jowls and turkey-necks. Lack of exercise makes the muscle tissue thin and wasted. Working isolated facial muscles with Facercise helps restore muscle tissue's elasticity and tone, making it plump and renewing strength. Like biceps, pectorals or abdominal muscles, facial muscles must be exercised in order to be firm, fit and strong.

Muscles are fibrous masses of tissue that are built of protein. Exercising muscles promotes the thickening and strengthening of muscle fibres. To strengthen a muscle, there must first be enough protein in the diet to ensure muscle growth. The goal of exercise is to make the muscle move repeatedly until it tires and the tissue breaks down: after this point rest is essential so the tissue can regenerate and grow bigger. It's really quite simple: the more a muscle contracts, the more it grows.

With the right balance of exercise and rest, the muscle adapts to the demands placed on it by growing bigger and stronger. Working a muscle to a heightened percentage of its capacity over a relatively short time will increase its size, strength and ability to contract. By isolating various muscles in the face and performing a repeated range of movements, the muscles are strengthened, regenerated and enlarged.

You may have heard of – or already tried – other facial exercise programmes. Facercise is unique and distinguished by its basic understanding of how muscles work. I've investigated some of these programmes; they'll instruct you to do things like open your eyes wide, stick out your tongue and hold this pose for ten seconds – without any logical explanation of how these bizarre methods work!

Uninformed programmes like these are as useless as those 'fat reducing' vibrating machines of the 1950s. Remember those? They had belts that you strapped around your waist so that you could magically jiggle away unwanted pounds.

No one who is truly interested in building their body would subscribe to this or any other get-fit-quick method. In these health-conscious times, we've become sufficiently aware of what steps need to be taken if one wants to reduce body fat and build muscle – a low fat diet, an aerobic exercise programme and a carefully applied routine of strength training.

Most of us know that exercises with weights or resistance should be done in multiple sets of eight to twelve repetitions in order to build size and strength. 'No pain, no gain,' has become an international exercise motto and, thanks to Jane Fonda, we've all learned to 'feel the burn' of working our muscles to the maximum.

Facercise is the first exercise programme to apply these same tech-niques to the face. When Facercising, you 'pump' the muscles around your eyes, for example, the same way you pump iron to develop a more defined chest, a shapelier back or sculpted arms. Personal trainers talk about the shape, size and definition of a muscle group; I'm encouraging you to think about the muscles in your face in similar terms.

Isolating and working muscles in the face to the point of feeling a lactic acid burn is the principle behind Facercise. This tingling or burning sensation occurs in a muscle when it is worked to capacity. The muscle produces lactic acid as a result of expending energy and using up ATP (adrenosine triphosphate), what exercise physiologists and personal trainers call the 'energy molecule'. Feeling the lactic acid burn tells you that you are making muscles grow stronger and larger.

In the eleven years that I've been teaching, I have consulted plastic surgeons in order to refine the exercises and make them as effective as possible. Doctors have confirmed my programme's safety and integrity, so don't worry that doing Facercise will overdevelop your facial muscles, a question I'm often asked by skittish exercisers. Facercise can only make you look and feel more attractive!

You may also be wondering if Facercise workouts may deepen wrinkles or stretch out your skin. Actually, the *opposite* will occur.

As you exercise, you increase blood circulation in the muscles and elsewhere in the face. The result is firmer muscles and taut skin with smoothed, less visible wrinkles. Although Facercise cannot restore lost collagen or elastin, neither can plastic surgery. (Collagen injections are painful and costly, can leave scars and must be administered every few months to maintain the puffy look. *Ouch!*) And, unlike plastic surgery, Facercise will greatly improve your skin tone from the inside out.

The programme in this book includes fourteen exercises that isolate about thirty of the fifty-seven facial and neck muscles. Because the facial and neck muscles are all interconnected by a network of fibres, every single muscle benefits.

Now that I've covered the basic principles of Facercise, I want to explain another reason why Facercise differs from other facial exercise programmes. Facercise involves more than performing a workout plan. One of the keys to its effectiveness is that it's the first facial exercise regime to harness two of your most powerful, renewable assets – your imagination and your energy.

Your mind and your energy play lead roles in making Facercise work. They work together to bring new beauty to your face in what I call the 'mind–muscle connection'. When I coach my clients, I tell them that they must *feel* their muscles working and *visualize* them growing bigger with every repetition. Devoting your mental and physical powers to these exercises is critically important to your success. You must visualize your muscles growing bigger and stronger with every effort.

Facercise's emphasis on feeling that burning sensation in the muscles is an indication of when you're doing the exercises properly. With such a powerful physical feeling to focus on, your mind stays on track, feeling the muscles grow as you work toward your goals. Your thoughts are as powerful as your actions, and if you *see* and *feel* your muscles enlarging and strengthening as you work, then your face will show the glowing results of your belief and effort.

So remember, when you do your workouts, I want you to be entirely focused on the mind–muscle connection. With these two allies, you can revitalize your face. Facercise provides more than short-term benefits: do your exercises for twenty minutes a day for at least five days a week, and you'll enjoy a life-long youthful appearance. Hundreds of my clients all over the world are living proof of this, and so am I. At forty-nine I can honestly say that my face is smoother, firmer, rosier and younger-looking than when I started doing Facercise at age thirty-six. And I've got the photographs to prove it.

BEFORE AND AFTER

The picture on the left was taken when I was thirty-six, pre-Facercise. My face was very wrinkled from years of sunbathing; I had wrinkles from the corner of my mouth to the middle of my jaw. I also had a thin, gaunt look because of collagen loss, another result of sun damage. My complexion was grey and not as rosy as I would have liked. My eyebrows were sagging and tired-looking, and my eyes looked small because the upper brows and eyelids were drooping so much. And no amount of make-up could conceal my under-eye bags.

From when I was twenty-one, my face wore the souvenirs of a bad rhinoplasty. My nose had a hollow on the left side and the surgeon had also left the nose tip too long so that it drooped downwards. In addition, the surgery had somehow made my upper lip descend and thin out.

Now take a look at the picture on the right, it's me, aged forty-nine, and it hasn't been retouched! The nasal-labial folds alongside my nose and upper lips have been smoothed out because the muscles underneath my skin are bigger and firmer. The wrinkles are less visible, and my skin tone has changed from grey to a porcelain, pink look. Facercising raised my eyebrows and toned my upper and lower eyelids, making my eyes look larger and more alert.

Thanks to my newly developed cheek muscles, my thin face has become fuller and more youthful-looking. My cheeks look firmer and rounder – it felt great to look in the mirror and see a new, sculpted, high cheek-boned face. (I can't tell you how many times people have asked me over the years, 'Who did your cheek implants?' When I tell them, 'I did,' they're confused until I demonstrate by pumping my cheek muscles for them *à la* Arnold Schwarzenegger!)

To my relief, Facercise made the dent in my nose invisible, and my whole nose looks and feels firmer. I also built up muscle in the nose (yes, there *is* muscle in the nose) so that the tip appears shortened. As for my lips, the upper lip no longer looks so low, and both lips have a fuller, more youthful shape. The corners of my mouth grew stronger and turned up for a younger, smiling, pert look. Another welcome change was a firmer jawline.

I always present these before and after photographs of myself when I go on television to talk about Facercise. Recently, I appeared on a television show and a woman who had tuned in called up to tell me, 'I saw your photographs and I don't think you look that different.' I replied, 'Well, thank you very much. Those pictures were taken thirteen years apart.' She signed up for instruction right there and then!

One of the most encouraging sensations of Facercise comes when you actually start to feel the muscles underneath your face. Suddenly you're conscious of that usually dead area between the cheekbones and the mouth, or the space between the ear and nose. Some clients say that after a few days of Facercise, brushing their teeth is about as painful as running up stairs the day after an advanced aerobics class. But they're happy because these minor aches make them more aware of their faces. They can feel that the exercises are working and are encouraged to know that their muscles are growing.

I take a great deal of pride in being able to offer such a healthy, easy and effective programme. And I believe that Facercise owes part of its success to the fact that people have fun doing it. Just imagine, by making faces for a few minutes each day, you can restore youth and vitality to your looks. An easy, enjoyable method for renewing your beauty, the exercises are also effective stress-busters that relax your face, body and mind.

FACIAL AWARENESS

How to pinpoint and understand your unique facial features

Any discussion of facial characteristics must also consider the nature of most women's self-image – especially your self-image. According to a 1994 article in *Self* magazine, 85 percent of women in the United States admit they don't like their bodies. Now that the global baby boom population is getting older, just imagine how many of them don't like their faces, either! What is your self-image like? How do you honestly feel about your face? Obviously you care about enhancing your appearance, because you're taking the time to read this book. If you're like my clients, you want to look as healthy and youthful as possible. And looking beautiful wouldn't be too bad, either!

But let's be realistic; very few people possess flawless complexions and beautifully proportioned features. Although heredity is the prime factor that determines your looks, and cosmetic surgery can dramatically alter your features, Facercise is going to help you improve your assets with an entirely natural method: the mind–muscle connection.

EXAMINE YOURSELF

Before you begin your exercises, however, it is critically important that you gain an objective, detailed understanding of your face. You may feel that you know your face very well – better than you'd like to at times! But I want you to be acutely aware of your naturally good features as well as your flaws. Most important, I want you to understand the circumstances that are behind whatever flaws you may have. Then, once we've studied your face in natural light, so to speak, we can start working on enhancing your looks.

I realize that studying your flaws and seeing how your face is ageing may make you uncomfortable. But it's the only way to begin. Film stars, models, rock singers, business executives and royalty have all submitted to this first step. If they can confront their flaws, then you can, too! No matter who you are, you owe it to yourself to assess honestly the beauty of your face. This way, instead of hoping for miracles, you can work towards realistic and positive improvements.

The circumstances of your daily life and your living habits directly affect your health and facial appearance. Stop and think about your environment for a moment. Do you live in a dry climate or a damp and cloudy one? Climate can have a detrimental or positive effect on the skin, as can the rhythms of your life. Are you always running on a tight schedule? Do you exercise often and take time to relax by yourself? Or are you too wrapped up in your career and social life to eat properly, sleep regularly and exercise? If you're stressed out and don't know how to renew your energy, this will show up in your face. Bags under the eyes, under-eye puffiness, pale or grey skin, wrinkles, frown lines and pimples – stress can cause all of these.

A photograph will show exactly what's happened to your face, how you really look, not how you think you look. So the best way to begin is to ask someone to take a close-up photograph of your face. Take two shots: front and side. Please do not smile! These photos will allow you to see your facial contours far more clearly than when you're looking in the mirror. And they will help you as you work toward correcting your flaws and allow you to observe progress as you go along.

These photographs are going to be especially useful to you in the future. Later on, after you have performed your exercises every day for a few weeks, you will take another two photographs from the same distance in the same head-on and side views. Then you can compare before and after and observe the wonderful changes that you have made in your facial features.

Study these photographs of your face very carefully. Every face – even a day-old baby's – has some lines. Without them, a face has no expressive quality. But what kinds of lines do you have? Are they thin or wide? Where are they most concentrated? Also consider how your living habits can affect your facial appearance. If you've spent years in the sun, as I have, then you probably have fine lines from all that suntanning. If you live on coffee, tea or fizzy drinks and rarely drink water to flush your system, this may account for blemishes, bags under the eyes or an ashen or yellow pallor. Drinking water is one of the best ways to keep the skin clear, rosy and smooth. You'll learn more about how diet affects the skin in Chapter 6, Your Skin Care Programme.

STOP WORRYING

Your emotional tendencies also have a great deal of influence over your facial features. If you worry a lot, this is bound to surface via lines in your forehead and/or around your mouth. Some people question things in their lives so frequently that they form what I call a 'question mark line' between the brows. Other people squint habitually, which leads to lines around the eyes.

It's also natural for people to store tension in their faces. Can you see where tension lies in your face? Many of my clients are still quite young, but because they have busy professional and family lives, they constantly look tense and drawn. Facercise can rapidly help correct this.

Although your personality, energy level and emotional characteristics influence how your face looks, heredity plays perhaps the biggest role in the formation of facial features and bone structure. It's odd how people's faces can age in the same manner that their parents' did. As I mentioned previously, a client will often come to me when her mouth starts looking like her mother's, or when his chin begins to soften like his father's. If you're in either of these camps, relax – doing Facercise can help play down inherited traits – but you'll have to work at it.

Continue studying the photographs of your face and zero in on

First Day: Dolly's cheeks are flat, she is developing jowls, and the combination of dull eyes, weak upper lip, and soft jawline give her a look of constant fatigue.

Sixth Day: Her face is more contoured, with higher, fuller cheeks and a tighter jawline. Her upper lip is more defined, and her eyes and overall appearance is more lively.

First Day: Sheila has a dull complexion, general lack of muscle tone, hollow under eyes, flat cheeks, a thin upper lip, sagging mouth corners, a heavy nasal labial fold and a double chin.

Sixth Day: Her complexion has become more vibrant, under eye hollows have faded, the cheeks are higher and fuller, the upper lip has filled out, and the mouth corners have turned upwards. With a disappearing double chin, her face appears more full, defined and healthy.

First Day: June's face seems dull, tired, and lacking in overall tone. She suffers from bags under the eyes, low and flat cheeks, a weak upper lip and a fleshy jaw and neckline.

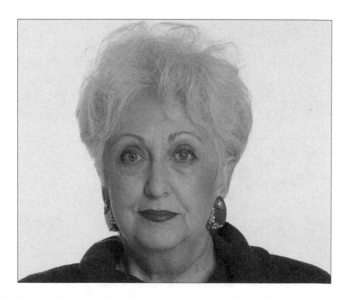

Sixth Day: Diminished under-eye bags, a more defined upper lip, and a tighter jawline and neck make her entire face appear healthier and more toned.

your best features and your least attractive ones. What feature do you want to emphasize? Your mouth? Eyes? Cheekbones? Which features do you want to play down? Your nose? Wrinkles? Double chin? Take another long, objective look at your face in the photographs and also determine your face shape. Is it long, round, heart-shaped? If you have full cheeks that are starting to sag in a round face, for instance, you can work at building them up with your Facercise programme.

THE TEN MOST UNWANTED FEATURES

1. *Thin hard-looking lips*
As you age, the lips and surrounding areas can become very thin and wizened. Tension, smoking, the sun and habitual facial expressions are the cause of this condition. The resulting lined and sunken effect can add years to your appearance and greatly detract from your beauty. The good news is that this situation can be visibly improved. My exercises will help rebuild the muscles around the mouth, giving a fuller, more youthful look to the face.

2. *Saggy jawline and/or double chin*
Even by the age of thirty or so, your jawline can start to sag, droop, and lose definition resulting in a weak, vulnerable 'grandmother' look. You can greatly improve the tone of your jawline by doing jaw-strengthening and neck-strengthening exercises. Another benefit you'll reap from doing jawline exercises is renewed confidence – many of my clients find that they speak more authoritatively after they've firmed up their faces and reduced their double chins.

3. *Low eyebrows*
When the muscle tone around the eyes weakens, the area under the eyebrows begins to look droopy and lowered, especially in profile. By doing an exercise that strengthens the eyebrow and scalp muscles so that the brow arch is lifted naturally, you will also strengthen the tiny but vital muscles in the eyelids and keep the entire eye area smooth and youthful. Practise this exercise with

dedication and not only your eyes, but your whole face will appear awake and alert.

4. Drooping eyelids

Take it from me – whether you're a drop-dead gorgeous movie star, a blue-blood aristocrat, or a fresh-scrubbed beauty, there's no escaping it: as you age, your eyelids start to droop. This can be a hereditary trait – drooping eyelids can run in the family. Besides giving the eyes a hooded appearance, the droops make you look older. You will learn a unique method of exercising the eyelids so that their mini-muscles become strong and the eyes open to become larger and more rounded. This creates a more wide-awake, vibrant look, and it will bring sparkle to your eyes.

5. Nose faults

It's very rare that you find someone who's perfectly happy with their nose, but let me tell you: large or small, long or short, noses grow larger as people grow older. As cheek muscles slacken and sag, a hollow area around the nose is created. While gravity pulls the nose down, the muscles around the mouth lose elasticity, which also contributes to the sagging. To keep your nose looking young and firm, the most important muscle to build up is the tiny nasal muscle located under each nostril. Exercising this area daily will improve the appearance of the nose as well as the tautness of the mouth and upper lip.

6. Crêpey neck

We've all seen people, even relatively young ones, with creased or crêpey-looking throats. This can be caused by too much suntanning, or poor diet combined with lack of exercise. And, of course, plain old ageing doesn't help the situation. Because the skin on the throat is delicate, it shows age more easily than other parts of the body. If your neck is thin and the muscles are not in tone, then the problem is compounded. On the brighter side, you can learn how to restore the shape and size of the neck muscles and thus improve the appearance of the entire throat area.

7. Flat cheeks

Gravity and age work together to flatten out the cheek muscles. As cheek muscles atrophy, the face begins to lose curves and flatten like a table-top. This casts a tired, older look over the face. The Facercise cheek-enhancing exercises can plump up the muscles so that your cheeks are sculpted and shapely. My clients love these exercises because they invariably help compensate for less-than-perfect bone structure. After doing these exercises for a few months, the resulting enlarged and strengthened cheek muscles will give your face a firmer, well-chiselled look.

By the time you reach your late twenties, your face is maturing along with your mind and body. All three affect each other and interact to form the personality that one presents to the world. Everyone has three different types of facial lines. By understanding how these lines differ from each other, you will be better able to work on correcting the damage.

8. Expression lines
Emotional reactions to all events and situations in our lives, such as sadness, anger and even joy, can be recorded in the face as lines – and these lines are not all bad, for they do give us our individual character. All of the Facercise exercises help plump up the underlying muscles of the face, which in turn smooths the skin out and diminishes lines.

9. Night-time furrows
Sleep lines are what I call the 'night-time enemy'. Your face muscles are working even while you sleep, smiling, frowning, etc. Sleeping with your hands lying under your cheek or burying your face in a scrunched-up pillow will cause cheek furrows. The cheek exercises will help smooth out the lines that are etched in your face as you sleep.

10. Wrinkles due to loss of muscle tone
The stomach isn't the only part of the body that sags as one grows older. The facial muscles also collapse if they are not properly exercised, and this causes the formation of lines. As we age and lose muscle tone and collagen, the pull of gravity loosens the skin and creates scalloped jowls and lines. Doing regular Facercise will help improve the general tone of all your facial muscles.

CHECKLIST FOR CHANGE

Now that you've considered the pros and cons of your facial features, it's time to get organized. Fill in the following checklist, ticking those features you want to improve. Now you have a record of what you are going to correct with Facercise. Later, you can compare your exercise results with 'before' and 'after' photographs.

    — Thin, hard-looking lips
    — Turned-down mouth corners
    — Saggy jawline/Double chin
    — Low eyebrows
    — Drooping eyelids
    — Long, flabby or enlarged nose
    — Crêpey neck
    — Flat cheeks
    — Expression lines
    — Night-time furrows
    — Wrinkles due to loss of muscle tone

Now you have studied your face in close-up and filled out the checklist you've earned a rest. Take a few minutes to reflect on all the changes that you're going to make in your face, and don't worry if you ticked every item here; you are not alone!

THE MUSCLES OF THE FACE:

Where they are, what they're called, how they work

By now you've committed yourself to making certain changes in your face. With this commitment, you *can* and *will* gain a more youthful-looking appearance. You're almost ready to get started. But first you need to understand where all your facial muscles are, what they're called, and how these small, interconnected units move. Picture this: beneath your skin, fifty-seven muscles are 'wired' together constantly, in motion and at rest. All these muscles rely upon each other to support and uplift your face.

Every time you smile or frown, several muscles team up to form your expression. For instance, the mouth and cheek muscles work with muscles around your eyes and temples when you smile. When you get tense, your scalp muscles work in tandem with muscles around the eye, and so on.

You may be wondering what this mass of facial muscles looks like. Imagine a magically moving patchwork quilt lying just beneath the surface of your skin. This thin layer of facial muscles is connected by bundles of fibres. I call these muscles magical because of the artistic feats they perform: working with connective fibres, they help express what you feel inside. Without the facial muscles and connective fibres, your face would look like a blank page.

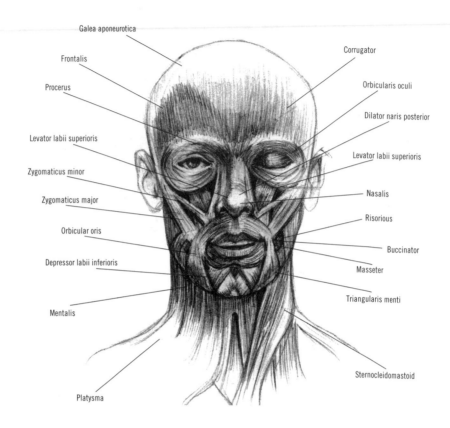

Facercise targets about thirty muscles in the face, neck and scalp. When developing my programme, I isolated these muscles because they decisively influence facial expression and beauty. I want to stress, however, that all fifty-seven facial and neck muscles are interconnected, so they *all* benefit from Facercise.

When you learn Facercise, it is vital that you practise the exercises as they are numbered, lesson by lesson. To gain optimum results, you *must* do the exercises in the sequence that they are presented. Why? Because while you're working one set of muscles, you want others to be resting and rebuilding.

Knowing where the various muscles are in the face, visualizing their ranges of motion and what their jobs are will help you make the crucial mind–muscle connection. If you can get into this state of mind/body, then you're sure to see good results in your face.

The ability to visualize and feel different muscles moving and growing as you work will help you do the exercises perfectly. And, as you work out, your muscles become so accustomed to their special movements that the exercises gradually become more effective. Take a few minutes to study the following description of your muscles and locate them on the illustration opposite. Knowing where your muscles are and what they do will help you bring your best face forward.

MUSCLES OF THE SCALP

You may be interested to know that the skin on the scalp is the thickest skin on the body. Underneath this skin, scalp muscles are divided into three areas:

FRONTALIS is a thin muscle located over the forehead. It draws the scalp forward, producing horizontal wrinkles in the forehead. *OCCIPITALIS* is about an inch and a half long and lies at the back of the head. It pulls the scalp backward. The occipitofrontalis (these two muscles together) is also known as the epicranius. *GALEA APONEUROTICA* is a broad, flat tendon underlying the scalp, joining the frontalis and occipitalis muscles.

MUSCLES OF THE MOUTH

ORBICULARIS ORIS completely encircles the mouth. It consists of numerous strands of muscle fibres, which go in different directions and connect with fibres in the upper and lower lips, cheeks, nose, and the surrounding areas. The *BUCCINATOR* is a broad, thin muscle beneath the cheek. It works to compress the cheek, as when you forcefully exhale or whistle. *MENTALIS* is a tiny muscle in the front of the chin which raises the chin and pushes up the lower lip. *QUADRATUS MENTI* is a small four sided muscle. It draws down the lower lip. Containing much fat intermingled with its fibres, this muscle benefits from exercise by making the lower lip look fuller. *TRIANGULARIS MENTI* is a triangular-shaped muscle rising from the lower jaw up to the mouth. It helps draw down the corners of the mouth. *RISORIOUS* is a narrow bundle of muscle fibres that retracts the corners of the mouth towards the back teeth. *ZYGOMATICUS* major and *MINOR* are two muscles comprising slender cords of muscle fibres that raise the corners of the mouth and extend into the cheek. They are also known as the 'laughing muscles' for the role they play when you smile. The fibres of the thin muscle *LEVATOR LABII SUPERIORIS* converge in the upper lip. The *QUADRATUS LABII SUPERIORIS* is a large muscle that lies around the upper lip and is connected to muscles in the cheek. The *PTERYGOID INTERNUS* works in tandem with other muscles to close the mouth and move the jaw. Exercising this will help create a well-toned jawline.

MUSCLES OF THE NOSE

Spanning the bridge of the nose, *PYRAMIDALIS NASI* draws down the middle of the eyebrows and wrinkles the nose. *DILATATOR NARIS POSTERIOR* is a small muscle situated above and behind the nostril. Working this muscle can help recontour your nose. Thin and delicate *DILATATOR NARIS ANTERIOR* lies directly above the middle of each of your nostrils. This is the muscle that causes your nostrils to flare. *DEPRESSOR ALAE NASI* extends across the base of the nose and closes the nasal opening by pulling down the septum, the cartilege partition between the two nasal passages. *COMPRESSOR NASI* begins at the bridge of the nose and extends up over the bridge, compressing the nostrils.

MUSCLES OF MASTICATION

These are the muscles used in the opening and closing of the jaws, for example for chewing and yawning. Many people hold tension in their jaws, and knowing where these muscles are and how to work them can help you relax, as well as build up muscle tone in the face.

The *TEMPORALIS* is a large muscle on the side of the head that closes the jaws with force. It goes diagonally back from the cheekbone to the outer jaw hinge. A short, thick muscle, the *MASSETER* also works in conjunction with the temporal to clench the jaws. Working this muscle helps firm up slack jawlines and double chins. The *EXTERNAL PTERYGOID*, short, thick and cone-shaped, helps to close the mouth and rotate the jaw. The *DIGASTRICUS*, what I refer to as the 'double chin' muscle, runs from the chin into the top of the neck. This serves to open the jaw.

MUSCLES OF THE EYE

The *LEVATOR PALPEBRA SUPERIORIS* in the upper eyelid is extremely thin but vital to maintaining firm, toned upper eyelids. The *ORBICULARIS OCULI* is a powerful muscle that surrounds the orbit of the eye. You couldn't see much without it, as it acts to open and close the eye. And you couldn't look surprised without it, because it helps to raise your eyebrows! When you squint, it raises the lower eyelid. The CORRUGATOR muscle juts out from the top of the forehead and runs into the muscle within the upper eyelid. Building this one can help smooth out forehead lines. The EPICRANIUS raises the eyebrows. Working this muscle helps increase oxygen and blood circulation throughout the forehead and eyes. Exercising the epicranius can also soften these brows, making you look more relaxed.

MUSCLES OF THE NECK

The PLATYSMA is a broad, thin plane of muscular fibres lying beneath the skin on each side of the neck. A powerful muscle, it produces wrinkles in the neck and also works to depress the lower jaw. The STERNOCLEIDOMASTOID rotates the head and draws it to either side. The TRAPEZIUS lies at the back of the head and shoulders and draws the head back and from side to side.

MUSCLES OF THE EAR

The following three muscles lie immediately underneath the skin around the ear. Although they have relatively little influence on facial appearance, these muscles are connected to the muscles that you work while Facercising. Most important, learning how to make these muscles move will help strengthen and define your scalp and face muscles. When you're doing exercises that firm your jawline, for instance, think about flexing your ears – this will help you work the jaw muscle group. Also, when you're doing exercises that lift and tone the upper eye and eyebrow area, flexing the ears will help lessen frown lines around the eyes.

The ANTERIOR AURICULARIS is the smallest ear muscle. Thin and fan-shaped, it draws the ears forwards. The SUPERIOR AURICULARIS, the largest ear muscle, raises the ears. The POSTERIOR AURICULARIS draws the ears backwards.

Now that you know the names and locations of various muscles, you're ready to start working them à la Facercise. You now possess both the vehicle and the map that will help you attain a more beautiful appearance. After you have read the exercises in the following chapter, you can begin your journey to a beautiful face.

THE EXERCISES

How to succeed at Facercise

The Facercise programme teaches you new skills that are gradually perfected through daily practice. Once you've memorized the fourteen exercise movements, doing them becomes second nature. After a few months of daily workouts, you will be experienced enough to start doing advanced versions of the exercises. (At the end of this chapter is a section which explains how to do a modified version of Facercise when you're driving.)

The great advantage of Facercise is that it's a flexible programme you can do anywhere or anytime. I Facercise throughout each day – when I'm talking on the phone, studying a menu in a restaurant, doing housework or watching television. As you learn the exercises in this chapter, you'll find how easy it is to work Facercise into your day, no matter where you may be.

As with all health and fitness programmes, it is essential that you schedule Facercise into your daily life and establish the right routine from the very start. I suggest doing the exercises in the morning for eleven minutes and at night for eleven minutes. To obtain the best results, you must do each of the exercises every day, twice a day, while you are learning them – and for six to eight weeks thereafter. Remember, good Facercise habits will help you recontour and tone your face quickly.

Most of my clients find that after a few months of disciplined workouts, they've knocked anywhere from five to ten years off their appearance. And believe me, people will begin to notice. There are no shortcuts in Facercise but, as I've said before, the exercises are fun and totally portable. Once you achieve the changes that you were seeking, however, you may advance to a 'maintenance' programme. This means doing your exercises every other day – or as your face needs them.

Got all that? Good. Store it in your memory bank. Now I want to wish you the best of luck with Facercise, and give you a gentle reminder. Get familiar with Facercise methods by reading through *all* the exercise directions two or three times before starting the programme. While you read, visualize and practise doing the exercises. You'll soon be on your way to a more radiant, youthful face.

A NOTE ON MY EXERCISE METHOD

One of the basic premises of Facercise is that you focus on the muscle as you work it to the point where you feel a lactic acid burn. The fingers or fingertips are often placed on top the muscles of the face to function as counterweights – the weight of the fingers provides resistance. This makes muscles work hard and grow bigger and stronger as quickly as possible.

Another exercise tip is to feel and visualize the energy that flows through your muscles as you work. When you read the exercise instructions that follow, you will see I often say things like, 'Follow the energy in your face.' My concept of energy flow is based on Traditional Chinese Medicine's theory that energy moves in pathways throughout the body. I also believe that there is an energy field around your body. Feeling and visualizing energy flows and energy fields helps people learn and memorize the exercises more quickly. Visualizing energy leads to more rapid muscle development than exercises done without involving your imagination.

When I mention energy and energy flows in the exercise instructions, I also often tell the exerciser to 'pulse' the fingers or make pulsing motions. By pulse, I mean making a rapid up and down movement. Pulsing helps you feel and see energy and perform the exercises correctly with maximum concentration.

FIGURE 1

Exercise 1

EXERCISE 1
EYE ENHANCER

RESULTS: The eye enhancer exercises the *orbicularis oculi* muscle that surrounds the entire eye. One of the most important muscles in the body, the *orbicularis oculi* opens and closes the eyes. This exercise pumps blood into the whole eye area and strengthens the upper and lower eyelids. It also reduces under-eye puffiness, lifts under-eye hollows and in effect enlarges the eye socket, giving you a more wide-awake, bright-eyed look. You may be wondering how the eye socket can be enlarged. Here are the facts: as you age, the upper eyelid muscle loses tone and sags down on the eye socket, invading the area and making it smaller. By toning and lifting upper and lower eyelids, the eye socket becomes enlarged and more defined.

METHOD: Do this exercise lying down or in a sitting position. Place your middle fingers between the brows, above the bridge of

FIGURE 2

your nose. Place your index fingers at your outer eye corners (Fig. 1). Make a strong squint up with the lower eyelid – feel the outer eye muscle pulse. Squint and release ten times, focusing on the pulsing each time you squint (Fig. 2). Now, hold the squint and squeeze your eyes tightly shut while counting up to forty. Focus your mind on the outer eye muscle pulsing. Be sure to keep eyes squeezed very tightly shut as you count.

REMEMBER: Do the Eye Enhancer exercise twice a day. Try it three times a day to correct deep hollows or severe under-eye puffiness, under-eye droop, or to enlarge the eye socket.

MEMO: In the morning, if your eyes are puffy and you haven't had time to Facercise, do two Eye Enhancers and then apply your make up. This will brighten your eyes considerably.

ADVANCED METHOD: After you have mastered the above exercise, try this one, which will bring you greater results faster. Do this exercise lying down. Each time you squint and release, lift your head off the bed or floor half an inch to make the muscle work harder. On the tenth squint, hold the squint and squeeze your eyes shut tight and count to twenty. Then raise head half an inch, continuing to keep eyes shut tight and count another twenty.

FIGURE 1

EXERCISE 2

LOWER EYELID STRENGTHENER

RESULTS: This exercise also strengthens the *orbicularis oculi*, firming the lower eyelid, diminishing the hollows under the eyes and reducing under-eye puffiness.

METHOD: This exercise may be done sitting or lying down. Place your index fingers at the outer corner of each eye, and your middle fingers at the inner eye corners (Fig. 1). Squint strongly with lower eyelids, thinking 'up'. Feel your outer and inner eye muscles flex (Fig. 2). Squint and release ten times, keeping your upper eyelids open wide. Now hold the squint and think 'up', maintaining the strong squint with your lower eyelid as you count to forty, focusing on the outer and inner eye muscles flexing. Repeat the entire exercise.

FIGURE 2

REMEMBER: Perform the Lower Eyelid Strengthener twice a day. If you have excessive under-eye puffiness, repeat three times a day.

ADVANCED METHOD: Do this exercise lying down. Each time you squint and release, raise your head half an inch off the bed or floor. Hold squint for twenty, then raise your head half an inch off the floor again and count for another twenty.

FIGURE 1

EXERCISE 3
FOREHEAD LIFT

RESULTS: This multi-purpose exercise works the *epicranius* which raises the eyebrows, the *frontalis* which draws the scalp forward, the occipitalis which draws the scalp back, and the *galea aponeurotica*, which joins the *frontalis* and *occipitalis*. The forehead lift prevents, or reduces, the frown lines between the eyebrows and raises the eyebrows. It also prevents or diminishes hooding of the upper eyelids.

METHOD: Try this in a sitting position or lying down. Place the index fingers of both hands high on the forehead so that they're parallel to the top of each brow (Fig. 1). Now pull the fingers down so that they're approximately half an inch above the brows. While

FIGURE 2

fingers are pressing down, concentrate on pushing the eyebrows up (Fig. 2). Push eyebrows up and release ten times. Now hold eyebrows in the up position, continuing to keep fingers pressed down – and do mini-eyebrow push-ups until you feel a tight band of pressure above the brows. Hold them up and count to twenty. Release.

REMEMBER: Do the Forehead Lift twice a day. It helps to clear the head and make you feel more alert. To correct a heavy or scowling brow, do it three times a day.

ADVANCED METHOD: Do the exercise lying down. Raise your head off the bed or floor half an inch each time you push up eyebrows and release. Feel the band of pressure across your forehead. On the final push-up, raise head half an inch and count to twenty.

FIGURE 1

EXERCISE 4
CHEEK DEVELOPER

RESULTS: The Cheek Developer exercises the *buccinator* muscle. This is the rounded top part, or 'apple' of the cheek. The exercise also works the *orbicularis oris*, which is the circular muscle surrounding the mouth. It lifts and enlarges the cheeks and removes hollows from under the eyes.

METHOD: Do this exercise in either a sitting position or lying down. Place index fingers on top of the apple of each cheek. Open your mouth and pull the upper and lower lips away from each other, forming a long, strong 'O' shape. Hold the long 'O' shape of the

FIGURE 2

mouth firmly in place. Keep the upper lip pressing down against the teeth (Fig. 1). Smile with your mouth corners and release (Fig. 2). Repeat thirty-five times, feeling the cheek muscles move under your index fingers. Use your mind–muscle connection and *visualize* pushing the muscle up under the cheek each time you smile. Your cheek muscles will really feel like they're working as you exercise. And after doing the Cheek Developer, your face will feel energized. REMEMBER: Perform the Cheek Developer at least twice daily. You can easily do this exercise while walking around the house or watching television.

ADVANCED METHOD: You guessed it this is another head raiser. Lift your head off the floor half an inch each time you smile and flex your cheeks.

FIGURE 1

EXERCISE 5
FACE ENERGIZER

RESULTS: The Face Energizer may sound similar to the Cheek Developer, but there is one crucial difference. The Cheek Developer makes cheeks fuller, but the Face Energizer uses the mind–muscle connection to combat the lengthening and flattening effects of gravity. The exercise works the *quadratus labii superioris* to work against gravity. It also helps remove the hard look of stress from the face and greatly increases blood circulation, giving your complexion a rosy glow.

METHOD: While lying down, pull the upper and lower lips apart, opening the mouth to form a long 'O'. Place index fingers on top of cheeks for light resistance, and keep your upper lip pressed down against the teeth (Fig. 1). Smile with your mouth corners and release feeling the cheeks move under the index fingers. Visualize pushing the muscle up under the cheek each time you smile. Repeat ten times. On the tenth smile, use all your strength to pull the upper and lower lip away from each other. Imagine your cheeks are moving out from the face and up toward the ceiling. Hold for a count of thirty. Take index fingers half an inch away from the face, then start to move fingers up in front of the face, towards the scalp

FIGURE 2

FIGURE 3

(Fig. 2). (This helps you move the energy field around the body as you *visualize* cheeks moving up through the top of the head.) Now raise your head an inch, hold it up and count to thirty while continuing to visualize (Fig. 3).

REMEMBER: Do your Face Energizer twice a day. If you're under stress, do it more often. An ache in your face is a sign that the muscle is getting stronger.

ADVANCED METHOD: Raise your head half an inch off the bed or floor as you smile and release. Repeat ten times, flexing the cheek muscles all the while. Continue the exercise as described above.

FIGURE 1

EXERCISE 6
NOSE SHORTENER

RESULTS: As I've said before, the nose continues to grow throughout our lives, and the tip drops and widens with age. The good news is that the Nose Shortener exercise shortens and narrows the nose tip by exercising the *depressor septii* muscle.

METHOD: In a sitting position or lying down, use the forefinger to push the tip of the nose up and hold firmly in place (Fig. 1). Flex your nose down by pulling your upper lip down over the teeth, holding for a second before releasing the lip (Fig. 2). Repeat thirty-five times, feeling the nose tip push against the finger each time. Remember to keep breathing at a steady rate while you do the

FIGURE 2

repetitions. This will aid your concentration as you work. Doing this exercise properly stimulates blood and oxygen flow in your upper lip and nose. Many of my clients describe feeling a tingling around the nose, which is a result of increased blood circulation. You'll feel relaxed and clear-headed after doing thirty-five repetitions of the Nose Shortener.

REMEMBER: Do the Nose Shortener once a day, twice if you're shortening a very long nose or narrowing a very wide nose.

MEMO: Some of my clients who have had rhinoplasty surgery report that doing this exercise for several weeks helps give their nose a more naturally sculpted look.

ADVANCED METHOD: Lying down, raise your head half an inch off the bed or floor each time while pulling down the upper lip and releasing it.

FIGURE 2

MOUTH CORNER LIFT

RESULTS: With age, the *zygomaticus* muscles sag, causing the mouth corners to droop. This exercise causes droopy mouth corners to firm up and turn up.

METHOD: This exercise can be done sitting or lying down. Close your lips together. Tighten the corners of your mouth into hard knots by sucking them in tight to your back teeth. Don't clench your teeth, and maintain steady breathing as you go. Place your index fingers lightly in the corners of your mouth (Fig. 1). Keep sucking the corners of your mouth in and *visualize* the corners turning up in a tiny smile, then *visualize* the corners turning down like a tiny

FIGURE 2

frown. *Imagine* turning them slowly up and down. Move your fingers away from the corners of your mouth in tiny up and down pulses, following the energy you feel in the corners (Fig. 2). Continue moving the fingers away until the muscles at the corners of the mouth burn. Hold the burn for a count of twenty moving the fingers up and down in half inch pulses. This will intensify the burn. REMEMBER: The success of this exercise relies heavily on your use of the mind–muscle connection. In your mind, you are visualizing the corner of your mouth going up and down about half an inch as you pulse the index fingers. This is a mental movement, not a physical movement! Do the Mouth Corner Lift exercise twice daily. ADVANCED METHOD: Raise your head half an inch off the floor or bed each time you visualize the corners moving up and down. When you feel the burn, keep your head up and count to thirty pulsing the fingers up and down.

FIGURE 1

EXERCISE 6
LIP SHAPER

RESULTS: By working the *orbicularis* oris muscle around the mouth, the Lip Shaper makes the mouth look younger, firmer and fuller. This exercise enlarges the lips and smooths out lines above the upper lip.

METHOD: This can be done sitting up or lying down. Close your lips. Don't clench your teeth. Put the tip of your index finger in between your upper and lower lips. Press lips together and visualize

FIGURE 2

your finger as a pencil that you are crushing (Fig. 1). Slowly pull your finger out from the centre of your lips while seeing and feeling the pencil. Draw the energy point out and lengthen your imaginary pencil until you feel the burn (Fig. 2). Pulse your finger up and down quickly for count of thirty.

REMEMBER: Do the Lip Shaper twice a day to plump up thin lips. This is a healthy exercise for people who hold their tension in their mouths.

ADVANCED METHOD: Do this lying down and raise your head one inch off the bed or floor as soon as you feel the burn. Hold, and pulse your finger quickly up and down to intensify the burn for a count of thirty.

FIGURE 1

EXERCISE 9
NASAL LABIAL SMOOTHER

RESULTS: This little workout can help make a big improvement to your appearance. By building up the *dilator naris anterior* and the *dilator naris posterior* muscles you will plump up deep creases and smooth out age lines from the nose to the corners of the mouth.

METHOD: This exercise works best when sitting in an upright position. Pull your upper and lower lips away from each other to open your mouth into a long 'O' (Fig. 1). Pull your upper mouth corners up into a smile – use only your upper lip. Wrinkle your nose

FIGURE 2

upward like a rabbit while smiling with the upper lip. Keeping your upper lip pressed against your teeth, push the upper lip down hard (Fig. 2). You will feel the pull along the sides of the nose. It's important that you wrinkle the nose up rabbit-style with each smile or curl of the upper lip – this forces energy to keep moving along the sides of the nose. Use your fingertips to trace and intensify the lines of energy along the sides of the nose up and down. Keep moving the energy up and down until you feel the burning sensation along the nasal labial fold. Hold the position, keeping your nose wrinkled, and quickly pulse the fingers up and down for count of twenty.

REMEMBER: Using your mind–muscle connection on this one helps intensify the burn and develop the muscle more quickly. Do the Nasal Labial Smoother twice a day, or more if your facial lines are deeply etched.

FIGURE 1

FIGURE 2

EXERCISE 10
NECK STRENGTHENER

RESULTS: This exercise strengthens the *platysma*, *sternocleido-mastoid* and the *trapezius* – all muscles of the neck. Besides helping to strengthen these important muscles that keep our heads upright, working them will firm up and smooth out the skin, counteracting sagging neck skin. After a few days of doing the Neck Strengthener, your neck will feel stronger, allowing you to hold your head higher. And this can help your posture – as well as your confidence.

FIGURE 3

FIGURE 4

METHOD: This exercise works best lying down. Grasp the sides of your neck under the ears with your fingertips. Press your fingertips into the neck (Fig. 1). Raise your head half an inch off the floor or bed, leading with the front of the neck, then lower (Fig. 2). Repeat twenty-five times, feeling how your neck muscles flex each time. Place your hands down at the sides of your body, lift your head and shoulders off bed, turn your head side to side, then lower back to bed each time before doing another repetition (Figs. 3 and 4). Repeat twenty times.

REMEMBER: Do the Neck Strengthener once a day if your neck is thick, and twice a day if it is long and thin.

FIGURE 1

E X E R C I S E   1 1
JAW STRENGTHENER

RESULTS: This exercise benefits the *pterygoid internus* muscle in the jaw. Working this muscle pulls up droopy jowls and erases sagging, scallopy skin around the jawline.

METHOD: In a sitting position, open your mouth and roll your lower lip in tightly over the lower teeth. Pull the corners of your mouth to the back and keep them rolled in like tight anchors. Keep your upper lip pressed against your teeth (Fig. 1). Open and close your jaw in a slow, scooping motion using the corners of your mouth

FIGURE 2

to open and close the lower jaw, imagining picking something up with your jaw as you scoop. Pull your chin up half an inch as you scoop. *Visualize* the sides of your face lifting up. Place your hands half an inch away from the sides of your face to help move up the energy field of the face. At this point, your head will be tilted back and your chin should be pointing toward the ceiling (Fig. 2). Scoop slowly and concentrate on visualizing the sides of your face lifting. After doing about six deliberate scoops, you should feel a burn. When you feel the burn, hold the pose and count to twenty.

REMEMBER: Do your Jaw Strengthener at least twice a day. Along with improving your appearance, it will also work to arrest further sagging.

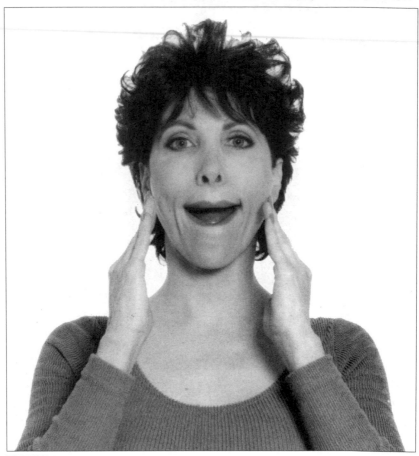

FIGURE 1

EXERCISE 12
FACE WIDENER

RESULTS: Especially helpful for long, narrow faces, this works several muscles and helps fill out sunken cheeks. It helps to widen the face and soften the thin, gaunt, 'witchy' look.

METHOD: You can do this sitting up or lying down. First, open your mouth and pull the mouth corners to the back teeth and roll them in like tight anchors. Keep your upper lip pressed down against the upper teeth (Fig. 1). *Visualize* big, fat cheeks coming out

FIGURE 2

of the corners of your mouth and filling in the gaunt area. Place your fingertips on your mouth corners and slowly pull fingers away from the sides of your face. Keep the corners of your mouth rolled in and pulled back (Fig. 2). Continue slowly pulling the fingers away until you feel the muscles burn, then raise your head about one inch. Hold it there and count to thirty-five. At this point, keep hands about two inches away from the sides of your face and make quick small circles with the hands to intensify the burn.

REMEMBER: The Face Widener should be done twice a day to correct a narrow or gaunt face. Skip this exercise if you think that your face is too wide.

FIGURE 1

EXERCISE 13
FACE SLIMMER

RESULTS: The Face Slimmer narrows, lifts and tones a wide face. Exercising the *buccinator* muscle will increase facial muscle tone. If your face is thin, do this exercise only once a day.

METHOD: Try this sitting up or lying down. Open your mouth and forcefully roll your lips over your teeth. Pull the corners of your mouth to the back teeth and roll them in like tight anchors (Fig. 1).

FIGURE 2

Use your mind–muscle connection and *visualize* the sides of your face moving up and out past the jawline to the top of the head. Place one hand on each side of your face, slowly moving hands up along the sides of your face as you visualize your face lifting (Fig. 2). Continue until you feel the burn. Hold and, if you're lying down, raise head one inch; count to thirty.

REMEMBER: Do the Face Slimmer twice a day if you have a heavy full face or for heavy sagging.

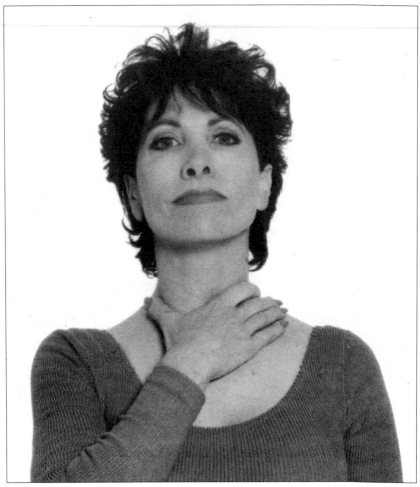

FIGURE 1

EXERCISE 14
NECK AND CHIN TONER

RESULTS: Great for firming the chin, neck and jawline, this exercise works and strengthens the *platysma* muscle. It can greatly reduce double chins and, in some cases, can make them almost invisible.

METHOD: Sit tall and straight with your chin held high. Close

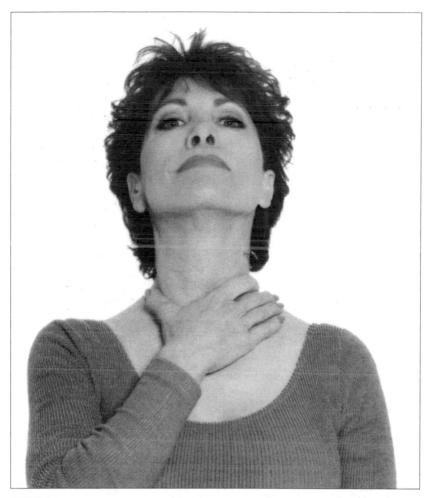

FIGURE 2

your lips and smile only with your upper lip. Place one hand at the
base of the throat over the collar bone and pull down slightly on the
skin with a firm grip (Fig. 1). Tilt your head back and release to feel
a strong pull on the chin and neck muscles (Fig. 2). Tilt head
backward then return to a normal head position thirty times.

REMEMBER: Do the Neck and Chin Toner more often than twice
daily if it is a problem area.

KEEP FACERCISING

Because I want you to reach your goals, I want to stress again that Facercise is a versatile improvement programme. You can fit your exercises in anytime, anywhere. These days, everyone's spare time is precious. Whenever you've got free time is the right time to Facercise. I've adapted the following exercises so that they can be done easily – and safely – while driving.

DOING FACERCISE IN THE CAR

My clients who drive say that they get quite a boost from doing Facercise behind the wheel. Along with making Facercisers look and feel more beautiful, the exercises help clear the head and improve concentration. Doing Facercise in your car may bring you other bonuses, as the following anecdote illustrates.

I had a client in her mid-fifties, who Facercised religiously in her car. One day, she was doing the exercises at a red light. When she arrived at her destination, a handsome man in his thirties pulled up alongside her as she got out of her car. 'Excuse me,' he said, 'I was driving behind you and I saw you smiling at me in the rear-view mirror at the red light.'

The woman laughed and explained that she had been doing facial exercises. He was intrigued, and when she told him her age, he couldn't believe it. He asked her to tell him more and at the end of their conversation, they'd made a date, despite their difference in age. So forget your self-consciousness and do your exercises in the car. Making the most of this time can yield unanticipated benefits.

All these exercises can be done whilst driving, except for the Eye Enhancer, which must only be practised when the car is stationary. Be careful to keep an eye on traffic lights and other vehicles – peek every few counts if you are squinting. **Do not endanger yourself or anyone else by Facercising while driving along, even at low speed.**

CAR EXERCISE 1 EYE ENHANCER

Place your middle fingers between your brows. Place your index fingers at your outer eye corners. Forcefully squint up with the lower eyelid – feel the outer eye muscle pulse. Squint and release ten times. Focus on the pulsing each time you squint. Now, hold the squint, and squeeze your eyes shut while counting to forty. Peek with one eye every few counts to check if the light has changed, and continue squeezing!

CAR EXERCISE 2 LOWER EYELID STRENGTHENER

Place your left thumb at the outer corner of the left eye and your left index finger at the outer corner of the right eye. Squint up and release ten times, feeling the outer eye muscles pulse. Hold for a count of forty, keeping upper eyelid open wide. Place your thumb and index finger at the inner eye corners. Squint up and release ten times. Then hold for a count of forty.

CAR EXERCISE 3 FOREHEAD LIFT

Place the thumb and index fingers of one hand on top of each brow across the forehead and pull your fingers down so that they're above the brows. Push your eyebrows up and release ten times. Then hold your eyebrows up, keeping the fingers pulled down, and feel the band of pressure across your forehead. Hold and count to twenty, whilst pushing away on the steering wheel.

CAR EXERCISE 4 CHEEK DEVELOPER

Place the thumb and index finger of one hand on top of each cheek. Open your mouth and pull the upper and lower lips away from each other, forming a long, strong 'O' shape. Keep the long 'O' shape of the mouth strong. Keep the upper lip pressing down against the teeth. Smile with your mouth corners and release. Repeat thirty-five times, feeling the cheek muscle move under your fingers. Use your mind–muscle connection and visualize pushing the muscle up under the cheek each time you smile. Repeat this exercise on the other cheek. You're pushing the muscle up under the cheek each time you smile. Repeat this exercise on the other cheek. You'll feel your cheek muscles pumping as you exercise and, as blood circulation increases as you work, your cheeks will feel energized.

CAR EXERCISE 5 | FACE ENERGIZER

While driving, pull the upper and lower lips apart, opening the mouth to form a long 'O'. Use the thumb and index finger of one hand on top of the cheeks. Smile with your mouth corners and release ten times, feeling the cheeks move under the thumb and index fingers. Imagine that you're pushing the muscle up under the cheek each time you smile. On the tenth smile, forcefully pull the upper and lower lip away from each other. Visualize pushing your cheeks out towards the windscreen, then up and out of the roof of the car. Count to forty. Slowly move your thumb and index finger off your cheeks, away from your face towards the windscreen and then up to the top of the car to help intensify the movement of the cheeks. Do this twice while on the way to an important meeting or a party. Your face will feel and look refreshed.

CAR EXERCISE 6 | NOSE SHORTENER

Use the forefinger to push the tip of the nose up and hold firmly in place. Flex your nose down by pulling your upper lip down over the teeth, holding for a second before releasing the lip. Repeat thirty-five times, feeling the nose tip push against the finger each time. Remember to keep breathing at a steady rate as you work. This exercise stimulates blood circulation in your upper lip and nose and helps warm up the face.

CAR EXERCISE 7 | MOUTH CORNER LIFT

Close your lips together. Tighten the corners of your mouth into hard clusters. Do not clench your teeth, and maintain steady breathing as you go. Lightly place your thumb and index finger on opposite corners of your mouth. Keep sucking in the corners of your mouth and visualize the corners turning up in a tiny smile and then turning down in a tiny frown. Pull thumb and index fingers away from the corners of your mouth towards the windscreen in small, up and down motions, to help you visualize the mouth corners at work. Continue to work the corners of your mouth until you feel the burn. Hold the burn for a count of twenty, pulsing the thumb and index fingers up and down.

CAR EXERCISE 8 | LIP SHAPER

Press your upper and lower lips together. Imagine you're crushing a pencil in the centre of your lips. Put your index finger between the centre of your lips. While pressing the lips together, pull it away slowly to the windscreen to lengthen the imaginary pencil. Push against the steering wheel with your other hand to intensify the resistance. Continue until you feel a burn in your upper lip, then pulse finger up and down for a count of thirty.

CAR EXERCISE 9 NASAL LABIAL SMOOTHER

Pull your upper and lower lips away from each other to open your mouth into a long 'O'. Pull your upper mouth corners up into a smile – using only your upper lip. Pull your nose up and wrinkle it like a rabbit while smiling with the upper lip. Forcefully push your upper lip down and keep it pressed against your teeth. You should feel the pull along the sides of the nose. Use your thumb and index finger to follow the energy up and down along the sides of your nose. Continue this movement until you feel the burning sensation along the nasal labial fold. Hold the position and pulse the fingers up and down quickly for a count of twenty.

CAR EXERCISE 10 NECK STRENGTHENER

The unusual method involved in this exercise provides excellent neck strengthening and toning results. Grasp the front of your neck with one hand as if choking yourself. Push your chin out away from your body, then relax. Repeat this action thirty times, feeling your neck muscles flex each time under your fingers.

CAR EXERCISE 11 JAW STRENGTHENER

Open your mouth and roll your lower lip in tight over the lower teeth. Pull the corners of your mouth to the back and roll them in tightly. Keep your upper lip pressing down against your teeth. Open and close your jaw in a slow scooping motion using the corners of your mouth, pulling the chin up half an inch with each scoop. Imagine picking up a long-stemmed flower using your jaw.

Visualize the sides of the face lifting up. Move one hand up in front of the lower face as you imagine that the sides of your face are moving up through the top of the car. Push against the steering wheel for resistance with each scoop. When finished, the chin should be pointing towards the top of the car.

CAR EXERCISE 12 FACE WIDENER

Open your mouth and pull the corners backwards to the back teeth. Roll in the corners of your mouth as hard as you can. Keep your upper lip against the upper teeth. Visualize big, apple-round cheeks growing out of the corners of your mouth. Use your thumb and index finger to make small circles away from your face to help 'pull' the energy out and fill in the gaunt area. Keep the corners of your mouth pulled back. Continue until you feel the muscles burn, making fast circles with thumb and index fingers to intensify the burn for a count of thirty.

CAR EXERCISE 13 FACE SLIMMER

Open your mouth and forcefully roll your lips over the teeth. Pull the corners of your mouth backwards to the back teeth and roll them in tightly. Visualize the sides of your face moving up past the jawline. With fingers spread out, move one hand up the front of your face to help 'move' the energy up along the sides of the face. Move the energy until you feel the burn. Push away from the steering wheel. Hold and count to thirty-five.

CAR EXERCISE 14 NECK AND CHIN TONER

Sit up straight with your shoulders relaxed and your head held high. Close your lips and smile only with your upper lip. Place one hand at the base of your throat over the collar bone and pull down slightly on the skin with a firm grip. Tilt head back and release. You'll feel a strong pull on the chin and neck muscles. Tilt your head backwards and forwards to the original position thirty times.

(6)

YOUR SKIN CARE PROGRAMME

I believe in a natural, self-disciplined approach to beauty because it's the simplest and healthiest way for a woman to develop good habits and maintain her unique good looks. Doing Facercise regularly can help you gain a more youthful appearance, but this coupled with a daily, preventive skin care regime is an even more effective beauty formula.

Practising preventive skin care every day is absolutely vital if you want to maintain a glowing, youthful complexion. This holds true even if you're a teenager, for today's poor cleansing habits or failure to use sunscreen can lead to tomorrow's serious skin problems or wrinkles. Your skin is an external organ, and it's exposed every day of your life – no wonder it ages faster than any other organ.

Skin is highly vulnerable to various factors in the environment, especially the climate and air pollution. Internal environments also affect skin: if your emotional life is stormy, your face can look strained or tired. If you're under stress, not sleeping enough or not eating properly, it will show on your face. The skin requires regular attention and special nurturing throughout life to look its best.

A CRASH COURSE IN SKIN BASICS

The skin is composed of three layers, the epidermis, the dermis and the subcutaneous tissue, also known as the fatty layer.

The outer layer of skin, or epidermis, consists of dead and dying cells which are constantly flaking off and being replaced with new ones arising from the base of the layer. New cells appear on the epidermis every twenty-eight to thirty days, but the cycle can be accelerated by conditions such as sunburn, windburn, poor sleeping habits, harsh cleansing and skin irritations. Conditions such as these will affect the moisture balance in the epidermal cells and influence skin texture. The epidermis can be fed and nourished through careful skin cleansing, toning and moisturizing.

Containing blood vessels, hair follicles and nerves, the dermis layer is also home to collagen and elastin fibres, and two essential skin glands. These are the sebaceous and the sweat glands. The sebaceous glands secrete an oil called sebum. When this substance is produced in excess, the skin erupts in pimples. The sweat glands secrete water and salts. The oil and water created in the dermis form an emulsion that protects and lubricates the epidermis. This emulsion also prevents oil and moisture loss, thus helping normalize the acid (pH) balance of the skin.

Collagen and elastin diminish in production as we age. This causes the connective and supporting tissues in our skin to sag and become slack. Sagging combined with lack of oil and moisture causes lines, furrows and wrinkles. If the dermis is under-nourished and has poor blood circulation, toxins may get stored in skin, causing the sebaceous glands to produce excess oil, which means eruptions on the epidermal layer. The condition of the dermis decisively influences skin tone and contours.

The third and innermost layer is the subcutaneous tissue, which is the fatty yet firm foundation of the skin. Acting as an internal cushion, the subcutaneous layer protects organs and deep tissues from the bumps and blows of daily life while insulating against the loss of body heat.

We are all born with normal skin, but genetics and hormones – two factors beyond our control – determine our complexions as we get older. But you can improve the condition of your skin through a healthy, positive lifestyle, good nutrition, exercise and dedicated skin care habits. Taking good care of your body and mind is the master key to looking good – and maintaining healthy skin.

The largest and most visible body organ, the skin is nourished by blood. Sleeping well, eating nutritious foods and increasing the flow of the blood to your outer skin tissues by exercising increases blood circulation and enhances the health of your skin.

As you know by now, the skin is shaped by bone structure and underlying muscle tissues. But it's also moulded by protein-based connective tissues which contain collagen and elastin, two substances which diminish in production as we age.

Collagen and elastin are fibrous strands that help make skin supple and plump. (Have you ever seen a woman who's had collagen injections in her lips? These injections give the lips a full, 'bee-stung' shape.) Elastin helps connect and support the skin: its elastic qualities help create supple skin tone. A diminishing supply of collagen and elastin in ageing skin is what causes it to sag. Collagen injections and implants are very costly, temporary treatments. Since collagen and elastin can never be naturally restored to ageing skin, all exercise, especially facial exercises, can help compensate by building up the underlying muscles, thus greatly improving the strength and beauty of your skin.

A literal bodyguard, your skin serves as a barrier against the sun's dangerous radiation and filters out dirt and toxins in the air. Just as a full-length mirror reflects your health, your skin registers your living habits and what kind of beauty care you practise. Because what you put inside your body dramatically influences how your skin looks, let's look at how and what you need to feed yourself to achieve a healthy complexion.

OXYGEN

From the moment we're born we must breathe in oxygen from the air or we'll never survive. Apart from being the essential vehicle for the production of usable energy, oxygen is also the body's personal assistant. It works around the clock, helping synthesize fats, proteins, carbohydrates and other substances in our food that help build and maintain cells, organs, muscles, bones – and all other bodily structures.

Having a good oxygen supply is an essential requirement for building a healthy body, mind and skin. Although some people use air purifiers in their home and office to improve the quality of the air they breathe, a mechanical purifier will never benefit your skin as much as regular exercise will – the most effective way to clear your skin through increased oxygen intake is to exercise at least three times a week. Perhaps you've noticed a healthy flush all over your skin after you've worked out – this glow is the result of increased blood circulation, a byproduct of high oxygen intake.

Clinical research studies conducted in various countries have proved that regular aerobic exercise – exercise that involves elevating your heart and breathing rates to higher than average levels for twelve minutes or more, three times a week or more – keeps you healthier, fitter and more relaxed.

Physical activity greatly benefits the skin by increasing the flow of blood throughout skin tissue, bringing oxygen and other nutrients needed for maintenance and repair of skin cells. Oxygenated blood helps process toxins and internal pollutants that damage skin and connective tissues. By exercising hard enough to make your skin flush, you can see how blood is circulating vigorously throughout your body.

If you're not athletic, even mild exercise, such as twenty minutes daily of brisk walking, will help get your blood pumping and your complexion blooming. In either case, it's always wise to get your doctor's approval before starting an exercise programme.

Deep breathing is also a mild but effective form of aerobic exercise and, like Facercise, you can do it anywhere. Even as you drive, sit at your desk or do the housework, deep breathing can make your body pump more blood everywhere, from your brain to your feet. Like an internal massage, deep yogic breathing gives you a calm but energized feeling.

Most of the time we breathe shallowly, using only our upper lungs. Deep breathing means breathing from your lower lungs, using the diaphragm.

Here's how you do deep breathing: sit up straight with shoulders relaxed. Do not lean forward. Inhaling through your nose, slowly fill your lungs with a deep breath. Expand your stomach area as you inhale, moving your diaphragm downwards. You should feel the air moving into the bottom of your lungs and then into the upper lungs. When you've reached maximum breathing capacity, hold the breath for one second, then slowly exhale through your mouth. Relax and breathe normally for four breaths. Repeat this process ten times. Deep breathing is a healthful and effective way to increase your energy and clear your skin. I urge you to practise this method whenever you can.

WATER

Your body needs water more than any other liquid. Drink eight or more glasses a day in addition to the other fluids you take in. This helps your body eliminate impurities, which leads to clearer skin. In addition, water helps reduce puffiness around the eyes and control hunger by making you feel fuller. Maintaining a healthy water balance is especially important for women. Drinking eight or more glasses of water a day can help you reduce premenstrual puffiness. Bottled mineral water or filtered contains less toxins than tap water. (Only reverse osmosis filters remove chlorine and other impurities from water. Get one of these for your kitchen and you'll have a high quality water supply.)

DIET

Proper nutrition is a vital part of the Facercise programme. We can't eat an imbalanced diet, such as one high in fatty, salty and sugary foods and expect to have the strength and enthusiasm to work at changing our facial contours through Facercise. To build strong, supportive facial muscles with a fabulous clear complexion, plus slow down the ageing process, you'll have to choose what you eat and drink with care. You are what you eat – and you'll look it!

We've all read and heard about various diets that are said to promote clear skin. But everybody's chemistry is different. The only way to learn what kind of vitamins and minerals your body and skin needs is to have a nutritionist take a blood sample and send it to a laboratory for a detailed analysis. Although it's impossible to recommend any specific diet, here are a few skin-friendly guidelines to keep in mind when making food choices.

Eating a diet that's low in meat and cheese and high in fresh fruits, vegetables and grains is a great way to feed your skin. Meats and cheeses are high in fat and protein and are difficult to digest. Animal products stimulate mucus production in the body, causing puffiness. On the other hand, the vitamins and minerals in fresh fruits and vegetables help build and repair cells. Many nutritional studies support the finding that vitamins such as Vitamin A, C and

E plus minerals like selenium and zinc combat the breakdown of collagen and elastin, your skin's supporting and connective tissues.

When it comes to dietary no-nos, salt is very high on the list. Salt makes you retain water and can make your face, and the rest of your body, look more puffy. Never add salt to your food. Instead, use herbs and spices if you crave extra flavour. Remember that there is enough salt in a balanced diet to satisfy your body's requirements.

Because it promotes water retention, drinking alcohol is one of the surest ways to make your face look puffy. And apart from containing lots of calories, alcohol also dehydrates your skin. If you do drink, do so in moderation. And drink a glass of water for every one of alcohol you imbibe. Water can help your body metabolize and excrete the alcohol more efficiently.

As for sugar, beware! Although it initially gives you a rush for twenty minutes or so, sugar is a depressant that can bring your energy level down. In the long run, the less sugar you consume, the more energy you'll have. Although nutritionists know that eating sugary foods is the surest way to gain weight through empty calories, it is unclear whether sugar intake causes pimples directly.

ANTI-AGEING SUPPLEMENTS

As for anti-ageing vitamin and mineral supplements, comprising antioxidants, there are many that have been clinically proven to protect the body from damaging free radicals. Free radicals are oxidants, or generators of toxic oxygen forms that cause molecular, cellular and tissue damage. Although free radicals can also be beneficial, most of the time they act like internal saboteurs, attacking other cells and contributing to the development of various health problems and diseases. The effects of free radicals not only age the cells in your body – they also make your skin look old, grey and lined.

Although free-radical activity occurs throughout our lives, these oxygen terrorists start doing serious damage when we're forty or older. Free radicals are most often ingested in rancid food or through polluted air. Air pollutants include nitrogen oxides, ozone and sulphur oxides. When inhaled, these substances generate free radicals.

If you smoke, or live with someone who does, realize that many of the toxic elements in cigarette smoke are oxidants.

Smoking is one of the most damaging things you can do to your body and skin. This is because cigarette smoke contains high amounts of nitrogen oxides, which happen to be free radicals! When they get in the body, nitrogen oxides can react with polyunsaturated fatty acids inside cellular membranes, causing rancidification, rigidification and death of cells. Clinical studies have shown, however, that vitamin E can help guard against these reactions.

Researchers established the cancer-causing potential of cigarette smoking decades ago. Many studies have concluded that free-radical activity is the primary cancer-causing factor in smoking. Non-smokers can also be affected by the toxic terrorists in cigarette smoke. I know smoking is a difficult habit to give up, but you can try. *Overwhelming* scientific evidence shows that smoking is unhealthy.

The most widely researched and used antioxidants include vitamins B12, E, C, A, folic acid and the trace mineral selenium. Beta-carotene and copper are also highly touted. Because everyone's biochemistry is unique, you should check with a nutritionist before going on an antioxidant supplement programme. Most importantly, no pregnant woman should take any vitamin, mineral, or food supplement without first consulting her doctor.

SLEEP

One of the most essential but most neglected ways to nourish skin involves sound sleep habits. Human beings are governed by natural biological rhythms, called circadian rhythms. In other words, it is more natural for people to go to bed before midnight and wake in the early morning than it is for people to go to bed at three in the morning and rise at noon.

International studies show that an overwhelming number of people are sleep-deprived. Make the effort to keep a regular bedtime – say 11 o'clock – and get at least seven hours of sleep each night. Your whole body, especially your skin, will feel and look more alive.

YOUR SKIN CARE HABITS

Now that we've covered internal skin care, let's look at how you need to care for the outside. Careful cleansing is the first step in any proper skin care regime. Dirt and dead skin cells need to be removed from the face in the morning and at night, possibly more if you exercise, have oily skin, or live in a polluted environment. Besides stimulating blood circulation in the face, thorough cleansing opens and cleanses pores. In addition, it helps prevent the skin's oils from clogging up and enlarging pores.

After cleansing comes moisturizing. After you cleanse in the morning, apply a moisturizer and then a sunscreen of at least SPF 30 to protect skin from ultraviolet radiation. (The sunscreen should be applied before your make-up base.) The more you are exposed to the sun, the more your skin will age. A suntan is actually the sign of skin damage, and if you want to safeguard against wrinkles, wear a sunscreen every day and stay out of the sun.

After cleansing at night, use a nightcream that will nourish and repair skin while you sleep. Eye creams are unnecessary if you're using a light but penetrating nightcream. The eye area lacks oil glands and the skin is extremely thin: heavy creams can actually weigh the skin down and promote wrinkles. Do yourself a favour and avoid rich, thick moisturizing eye creams.

No skin care regime is complete without exfoliation, the clearing away of dead skin. Regular exfoliation with a botanically based enzyme mask will get rid of the old and bring in the new. In my experience, the enzyme masks that work the best contain proteins RNA, L-Lysine and Proline. These cleanse and penetrate to tighten the epidermis. A good enzyme mask will constrict, tone and tighten skin while drawing out impurities from the pores.

The skin care products I find most valuable for all skin types are transdermal, meaning that they are so water soluble that they are actually stored in the skin for hours. Because they penetrate and rest inside the skin, transdermal preparations favourably influence the functions of cells and glands within the dermis. How can you find high quality transdermal products? Dermatologists and skin care salon therapists are the most knowledgeable sources for these. You may, however, find some good ones on your own. Be sure to read labels and check for 'transdermal' properties.

I have used various skin care products containing alpha-hydroxy acids (AHAs); many dermatologists and beauty therapists recommend these for their superior cleansing and skin-balancing properties.

Although controversial, the vitamin A derivative Retin-A does have its merits as an acne treatment. In the late 1980s, some researchers claimed that it could undo years of skin damage caused by ageing and suntanning. I have never seen this happen. Rather, Retin-A can smooth out fine surface lines – but that's about all. In addition, no one knows what the long-term positive or negative effects of this cosmetic pharmaceutical may be. However, there are indications that skin becomes over-sensitized to the sun, requiring a life-long use of sunscreens.

Some cosmetic manufacturers claim that new, oxygen-bearing emulsions can actually penetrate the skin and bring other nutrients, such as vitamins A and E, directly into skin cells for repair work. Refer back to the previous discussion of oxygen, the great vehicle for producing energy in the body. Oxygen-bearing cosmetics are some of the most highly touted products on today's market. The main active ingredient in oxygen cosmetics is hydrogen peroxide. Bacteria, which contribute to skin problems such as acne, cannot survive in an oxygen-rich environment. Hydrogen peroxide is readily reduced to water, giving up oxygen in the process. This causes frothing, which helps to dislodge dirt and dead skin cells. In addition, it acts as an antiseptic and deodorizer.

You can experiment on your own with oxygen-based treatments by pouring a bottle of hydrogen peroxide solution (3 percent) from the chemist into a plastic spray bottle. Spritz it on your face in the morning and you'll feel and look refreshed. I pour a whole eight-ounce bottle of solution in the bath after a long day and I feel as if I've had a full body facial. (A hydrogen peroxide solution bath is also a great remedy for jet-lag.) But be careful – full-strength hydrogen peroxide is a bleach.

Steam baths are another low-tech yet effective method for opening pores and cleansing skin.

BODY SKIN SECRETS

Although I use moisturizers on my face, I take a different view of how to nourish the skin on the rest of my body. This may sound sacrilegious coming from a skin care expert, but the best way to achieve soft, supple skin is by never using moisturizers on your body. I know I don't. Here's what I do instead: every morning before I take a shower or bath, I give myself a quick 'body facial' that hails from Baden-Baden, one of Europe's oldest and most renowned spas.

Use a *dry* sisal or loofah mitt. Put your right hand in the mitt and start on the sole of your left foot, making counter-clockwise circular motions – this stimulates blood flow in the direction of your heart. Circle up your left leg to the stomach, then make circular motions on the top of your left hand and up your left arm and breast. Now put your left hand in the mitt, and start on your right foot, repeating the pattern. Then with your hand in the mitt shimmy the scrubbing fibres up the back of your legs, buttocks, back and neck. Rinse the mitt in water once a week and allow to dry overnight.

By stimulating blood circulation and sloughing off dead skin cells, this daily treatment energizes you and helps eliminate toxins from the skin. Dry exfoliation promotes a healthy, pink glow and soft, fresh-feeling skin. Another benefit is that it's cost effective and can save you the expense of body lotion. A good quality loofah or sisal lasts several months.

NIGHT-TIME SKIN CARE SECRETS

Some people barely recognize themselves when they get up in the morning. This is because they sleep on their stomachs with their heads pushed into the pillow and they wake up with puffy areas and sleep lines that make them look tired and creased. You can avoid this situation by conditioning yourself to sleep only on your back, without a pillow under your head. Instead, put the pillow under your knees before going to sleep. You'll see the difference in the morning.

As I've explained earlier, we move our faces in sleep the same way that we do during waking hours. You frown and smile often during the day; you repeat these same expressions as you dream. To reduce lines in the forehead or between the eyebrows, apply surgical tape on skin furrows before going to bed. Try it for four nights in a row and you'll see that your skin looks smoother in the morning. I routinely tape the area between my eyebrows before going to bed as this helps smooth out the lines.

Let's face it: the only thing standing between you and beautiful skin is your mind. If you visualize how your eating, lifestyle and grooming habits will affect your looks, then you will behave carefully to achieve your beauty goals. Every method and tip discussed in this chapter can be easily integrated into your daily life.

Keep Facercising and remember to pamper your skin every day, morning and night.

In the eleven years I've been teaching Facercise, I've seen people of all ages and walks of life enjoy remarkable and healthy changes after devoting twenty minutes of their day to the programme. Whenever you need encouragement, take another look at Chapter 3's dramatic before and after photos. I've also included on the following pages some actual letters of testimony and thanks I've received from clients over the years. I promise you that by doing the exercises in this book, you too can give yourself a natural facelift.

Facercise has taken me around the world to teach people how to realize their inner and outer beauty. There is an old Chinese saying, 'When the student is ready, the Master appears.' Experience has taught me that many people on this planet are ready for Facercise. When I train someone and see how their face changes after doing the programme, I feel great satisfaction and happiness for them. Why? Because they did it themselves, and they feel and look terrific.

You, too, can revitalize your own unique beauty. If you want a more youthful and toned face, a rosier complexion, firmer skin and sparkling eyes, all you have to do is Facercise.

TESTIMONIALS

Dear Carole,

I'm so happy, I read about Facercise in *Harpers & Queen*. Your course was intense, fun and results quick coming. My lips are fuller and my nasal labial line is nearly gone. I continue to exercise my face in the car and really quite like it. Thanks for all your help.

Fondly,

Sue Gigins
New York, NY, USA

Dear Carole,

I'm writing you this letter on my 50th birthday to tell you how much enjoyment I have already received from my 'big gift', Facercise. Although it's only been four weeks since I completed my classes with you, my husband and family are thrilled with the results. My husband feels it's the best money he has ever spent on a present. I feel great and all my friends think I look years younger. The best part is that there is no doctor, no cutting, and no waiting months for it to 'relax'. My results were almost instant. Thanks for the new me.

Warmest regards,

Jane Miller
Scottsdale, AZ, USA

Dear Carole,

When I signed up for your course on facial exercise, I was sceptical. It has now been twelve days and I have had at least six clients and friends ask me what I was doing for my face because I looked really good.

I now have cheeks, larger lips and a wider face, something I thought was impossible with my features! I also have a problem with jaw-grinding, and I have noticed that the jaw exercises have helped relieve my pain and tension. Your programme is unbelievable and I can't thank you enough. It has really helped my confidence!

Best wishes,

> Joan M Lessner
> Redondo Beach, CA, USA

Dear Carole,

After eye surgery several years ago, I trained with you and your program and was pleasantly surprised to find my eyes wider and my face much stronger. Had I known prior to my surgery what your programme could do for me, I would never have undergone the surgery. I'm confident in saying to everyone that they should train the muscles in their face. This training has given me more confidence and personal satisfaction in my appearance.

Love,

> Jan Fuson,
> Redondo Beach, CA, USA

Thanks to Facercise and Carole Maggio I feel like a new woman!

Facercise is absolutely fabulous! I love the one-to-one training with Carole: she has introduced me to a new world of extensive facial exercises which have now become part of my daily routine. In only twenty minutes, whether I exercise at home or in the car, I feel refreshed and invigorated, knowing the results are truly rewarding.

I started the exercises a month ago and already have had many, many wonderful compliments on how I look. It had been a while since I had seen some of my friends and when we were recently together at a convention, they commented on how great and 'different' I looked. The 'difference' is due, of course, to my facial exercises.

When working with Carole during the face training, she took a photograph of me at the beginning, the middle and the end of the sessions. What can I say? The pictures said it all! The visible changes are absolutely remarkable, and all in just five days!

Facercise has definitely made me feel younger and more attractive. Thank you, Carole, and I LOVE YOU FACERCISE!

> Alexa Coon
> Washington DC, USA

Dear Carole,

I want to tell you how my progress has been since I took the Facercise course about three years ago. Remember I came to you really out of desperation, as I had exhausted all other obvious options. I wanted to get rid of my acute scarring and had had three dermabrasions already. My only other option, according to several plastic surgeons, was a face-lift, which most likely would have to be done every couple of years. Well, my results with Facercise have been beyond what I had hoped for.

My eyes, which were always half-closed, are more open and brighter. My acute scarring is barely visible because I've been able to pump my cheek area out. I always had pale, yellow, lifeless skin; my skin is now pink and much brighter. My husband, a medical doctor, was kind of doubtful about the course, but he was astonished by the results and has given me nothing but encouragement to share this with others.

Love,

> Laurie Ellen McGarry
> Carmel, CA, USA

Dear Carole

My mother taught me to write thank-you letters, but this is the first I have ever written for 'services rendered' and yet it is probably the most heartfelt of any.

As you may remember, I was quite sceptical of the value of face exercises when I read the article about you in *Longevity* and called you with a thousand questions. However I was desperate for help and mortally afraid of surgery, not to mention that the cost was way beyond my means. It was talking to three of your satisfied clients that finally convinced me to take the training.

Yes, I know, Carole, I was a difficult student, but you, against heavy odds, created a remarkable change in my face – well, really I should say you helped me create the change which makes me very proud of myself. What brought me to see the point of writing this thank-you letter was seeing my college roommate last week at a Pan Hellenic luncheon, and knowing me so well and feeling she could say anything to me no matter how outrageous, she popped out with,'My God, Nancy, who did your facelift? You look fabulous!' Wow, what a testimony to what you and I achieved together!

Thank you, Carole,

Nancy Cooksey
Monterey, CA, USA

Dear Carole,

I find myself at a loss for words to describe how I feel about your Facercise programme, as I'm quite certain your many clients are. So here goes! THANK YOU! THANK YOU! THANK YOU! You have a magical gift in the Facercise programme.

Six days ago I began the facial exercises. Many of my friends have had plastic surgery; some, to my horror, look as though they are wearing a tight mask. Their faces look different to me, not better. A close personal friend has no feeling in her left cheek – the surgeon says it may return in time.

I am a woman in my sixties and thought my only option was to take my chances and go under the knife. I heard about you and because of my fears, not because I believed a facial exercise programme would work, I came to you.

You are remarkable. My face looks youthful again, and the sag in my jaw and neck is improving. Just this morning as I was leaving the gym, two women asked me what I had done to my face – I looked much younger and radiant to them.

To think that six days ago I felt hopeless and even depressed when I applied my makeup. I thank God for you, Carole Maggio, and will send clients to you. I now am planning a trip to London with the $10,000 I saved by choosing you instead of the surgeon.

Sincerely,

Anne Bennett
Palos Verdes, CA, USA

Dear Ms Maggio,

You asked for an update of my physical progress after my sessions with Facercise. I am happy to report that the feeling has returned to my face, especially the right side. In addition, my face is fuller and the flatness has disappeared, just as you said it would.

My partner Paul is delighted with my progress; he was by my side during a long and painful ordeal with Bells palsy. Now he would like to schedule time with you.

Thank you for the healing and uplifting programme you've developed.

George TK
Chicago, IL, USA

FACERCISE PROGRAMME CALENDAR

Here is a Facercise agenda that you can use to keep track of your exercises in the crucial first month – and in the months beyond. Remember to do all of the exercises twice a day, or more, depending on your goals.

1. EYE ENHANCER
2. LOWER EYELID STRENGTHENER
3. FOREHEAD LIFT
4. CHEEK DEVELOPER
5. FACE ENERGIZER
6. NOSE SHORTENER
7. MOUTH CORNER LIFT
8. LIP SHAPER
9. NASAL LABIAL SMOOTHER
10. NECK STRENGTHENER
11. JAW STRENGTHENER
12. FACE WIDENER
13. FACE SLIMMER
14. NECK AND CHIN TONER

1	2	3	4	5	6	7
Facercised all 14 exercises	Facercised all 14 exercises	Facercised all 14 exercises	Facercised all 14 exercises	Facercised all 14 exercises	Facercised all 14 exercises	Facercised all 14 exercises
___ times	___ times	___ times	___ times	___ times	___ times	___ times
8	9	10	11	12	13	14
Facercised all 14 exercises	Facercised all 14 exercises	Facercised all 14 exercises	Facercised all 14 exercises	Facercised all 14 exercises	Facercised all 14 exercises	Facercised all 14 exercises
___ times	___ times	___ times	___ times	___ times	___ times	___ times
15	16	17	18	19	20	21
Facercised all 14 exercises	Facercised all 14 exercises	Facercised all 14 exercises	Facercised all 14 exercises	Facercised all 14 exercises	Facercised all 14 exercises	Facercised all 14 exercises
___ times	___ times	___ times	___ times	___ times	___ times	___ times
22	23	24	25	26	27	28
Facercised all 14 exercises	Facercised all 14 exercises	Facercised all 14 exercises	Facercised all 14 exercises	Facercised all 14 exercises	Facercised all 14 exercises	Facercised all 14 exercises
___ times	___ times	___ times	___ times	___ times	___ times	___ times
29	30	31				
Facercised all 14 exercises	Facercised all 14 exercises	Facercised all 14 exercises				
___ times	___ times	___ times				

CAROLE MAGGIO

About the Author

Carole Maggio is a skin care specialist who for eleven years has taught Facercise® to clients across the United States, Europe, the Middle East and Japan. She has conducted beauty seminars at the University of London, served as an instructor at one of Tokyo's foremost beauty establishments, and has lectured at conferences and before selected audiences around the world.

For information on audio cassettes and personalized instruction please send a stamped, self-addressed envelope to:

Carole Maggio Facercise
8485 East Macdonald Drive 328
Scottsdale, Arizona 85250
USA